BACK ACHE

Eliminate Back Pain, Realign, Repair & Maintain Your Spine

SAM RAO

First published in Great Britain by Sam Rao in 2018
www.samraoyoga.com

Acknowledgments

Book Publishing Services – Eleanor Hayes at Bookzang
Photography – Sarah Robertson

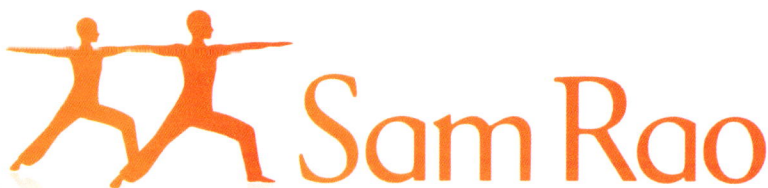

Sam Rao

YOGA · TEACHER TRAINING · WELLBEING

Contents

Preface

It is through fear (perception) and denial (reason) that one abrogates self responsibility to others for their health.

This book is dedicated to my teacher Dr Ben Carraway, who taught me not to fear and to take responsibility. I know that this story is one of the finest examples of no matter what, obstacles can be overcome.

Chapter One

My own story

My recollection of doing yoga goes back to when I was approximately 5 years old. My mother used to practise postures which I copied. My earliest recollection is of my mother, standing on her head, with her sari tucked between her legs. The sari had a blue wide band at the edge. She is talking to me about something.

Right through to my teenage years I remember doing various yoga postures…there was a time when the warriors appealed to me the most and then there was a time when my father taught me the art of Lathi. It is a way of using a 5ft long bamboo pole and learning to use it as in art of defence. Those years are clear in my mind. The whole body is used and the shoulders and arm muscles were the main focus. For a teenager that was the best pay-back!

Then I went on to Vancouver for my high school and university. I enjoyed the 1960s from 1963 onwards until 1971 when I arrived in the UK. I got married and have lived in the UK ever since. My yoga discipline kind of faded into the background of life of parenthood.

In the mid-1990s I had taken up squash and was regular at my local squash club, mainly playing for fun and for good exercise. I eventually got in to a competitive league and it was during 1998 and a particularly strong squash session (trying to remain high in the local league), that I suffered a damage to my lumbar spine. It was painful at the time but I kept on playing (mistake!) and I did not do anything to have the spine looked at, but did let go of squash and switched to other sports which did not give my spine any trouble. Yoga was once again entering my life and several teachers appeared as I became more and more interested in developing my yoga. My spine was not improving but it did help me to work with yoga postures to maintain the status quo, living with the pain and doing different sports when the spine was ok.

In 2001 I met my yoga teacher, Ruth White, and trained with her to become a yoga teacher. I was still not sure what I was going to do but I liked the idea of developing my yoga teaching skills.

I combined my software-selling business with teaching yoga in my local community and it soon became clear that there was a living to be made, a business to develop, from teaching yoga.

By the time I graduated in 2003, I was already teaching 2 classes a week and planning my business development plans for yoga. I had come to realize that I could not keep on going with the business of sales and software, which was just that, a business with no positive and enjoyable personal returns. Yes, I was making money but I wanted more, I wanted to work with people who were interested in looking after themselves but through yoga.

My yoga classes in Berkshire and yoga retreats in Greece developed enough for me to sell/wind-down my commercial business. Yoga became the main and the only source of income. It was a bit difficult to start with, but then I realized that when I was ready all that I needed arrived. I did not so much match my income to what I was used to, but adjusted my lifestyle to what I wanted and could afford to live well.

My local yoga classes, all my 1-2-1 clients, yoga retreats, visiting teacher trips to various parts of the world culminated in a wonderful way of living. I even experimented with moving to Monterey, California because of the number of students I had there during my regular yearly visits. For a very good reason the US Government decided that they could not afford me a visa to start building my business there. I say it was a very good reason because that opened my eyes to looking at my business in a different way.

My yoga business was and continues to be very successful, but my wish to increase my own learning/teaching prompted me to open my own yoga teacher training school. And so it continues to this day. Several full classes, 2 retreats per year, teaching 10 to 12 students to become yoga teachers. All in all, a thriving state of affairs.

During 2011–2012 I found that my spinal health was deteriorating. It was gradually becoming more and more difficult to walk long distances. I found that I had to squat down to release the sciatic nerve during my walks. The periods between walking and having to release the nerve got shorter and shorter. I sought medical advice and discovered that none of the doctors and consultants I came across could help me except to only offer drastic surgery.

In fact it took a while before I woke up to the fact that the people to whom I was being referred for a possible solution, almost all of them had some kind of problem with their own backs. So why was I going to people to get my back sorted, when none of them were well in their lower back?

I also needed to listen to my own inner voice and ask for help. I also knew, and believed, that through yoga I would be able to heal myself. So now I found myself in a lot of pain and really wanting to get better. The universe responded and within days an enlightened Chiropractor came in to my life. He was suggested to me by a distant friend whom I had not seen for many years.

I have dedicated this book to Dr Benjamin Carraway (Ben) who was the only "medical" person who looked upon my spinal issue with a completely different attitude. He examined me thoroughly, asked lots and lots of questions about my lifestyle and started to manipulate and treat my spine. The first visit was fine, not much improvement, but fixed a second and longer visit for next day. There followed lots of manipulation, but Ben did say he was working on locating the problem areas.

Ben saved the best part for the last 10 minutes. I remember him clearly saying at the end of this second visit: "Sam, I think we can fix this in six weeks".

Obviously this was music to my ears. Ben had seen a lot of back problems in yoga teachers and he did use yoga postures to help to correct spinal issues. My spine was in a dreadful state and I did share one or two of the images from x-rays and MRI scans to let Ben know that even from such a stage of deterioration, there is a way back. With precise guidance from Ben we worked out a programme to allow me, within 12 weeks from the start of treatment, to declare to Ben that my spine was in good enough shape for me to do a lot more of the walking and cycling, which I love. My spine was not completely back to normal and I knew that I had a year of hard work ahead of me.

This was my spine in 2011–2012 (see image, right). I had an MRI Scan and x-rays to confirm the level of deterioration.

A year later (late 2012) with daily practising of yoga postures that Ben had suggested, I was almost out of the woods. I had a routine of spinal check every 9 weeks with Ben. After about a year I finally heard Ben say during one of my regular check-ups that my spine had finally come back to its original alignment. In fact what had happened is that all the muscle structure around the spine had been developed to help brace and support the spine as it should be in normal spines.

Now, aged 68, I am as fit and as mobile as I was in my 40s and 50s and I continue to share my experiences of how to sort out a spinal problem with a wide range of my own clients.

When my 1-2-1 clients come to me to help them sort out their back pain problems, I get them to agree on 2 main requirements.

- One is that they agree and discuss with me that they are prepared to do what I ask them to do, in terms of their yoga postures and their diet (supplements).

- The second is that through our conversations I become aware and agree with my client that they really do want to get better. If there is no real desire to become well, then I do tell them and then let them go.

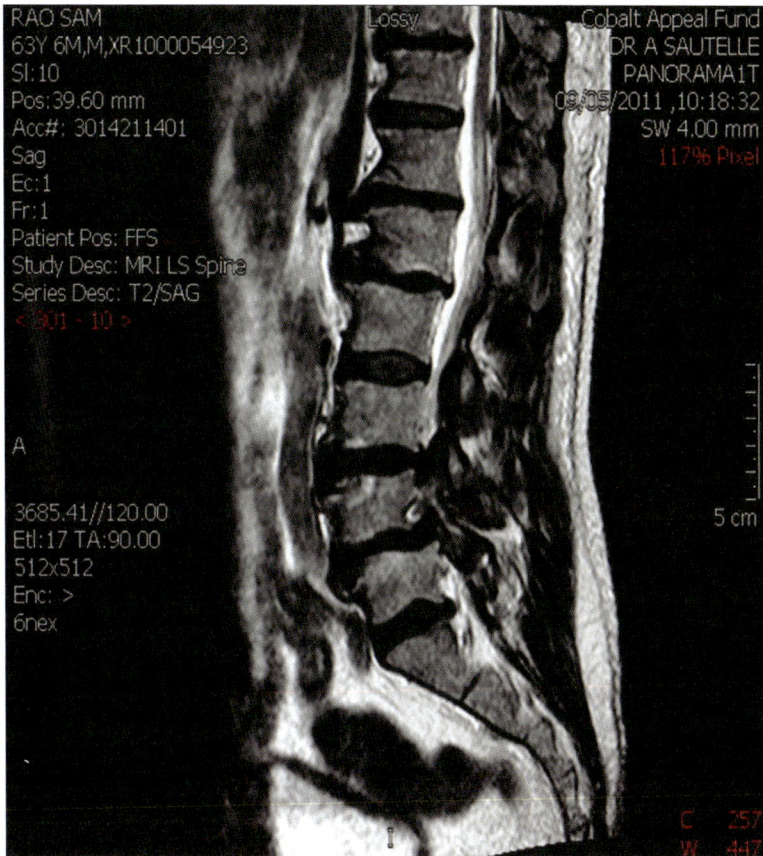

MRI SCAN 09-05-2011 Lumber 1 was pushed back Lumber 4 has a
stenosis & Lumber 5 is out of alignment with L4 and S1

Sciatic nerve was constantly being aggravated and required me to
squat down to release the pressure. A 2-page Consultant report stated,
through highly complicated words, which I have simplified for myself.

1 L2 was out of alignment with L3 and slipping towards my left side.
2 L3 and L4 were squashing together and "opening inwards".
3 A stenosis between L3 and L4 which means the spinal cord was
coming out on the inside, towards my pubic bone. That led to exposed
nerves which were irritating the area.

Proof that the spine in this area was getting worse and consequently I
was getting the pains when I walked.

That there is an increasing number of people with health issues is not new news. Everyone is aware that there is a growing trend of a wide range of conditions that require more and more resources to put them right. The NHS is already overloaded. The pharmaceutical companies are thriving, the number of people living with a range of supports (wheelchairs, motorized chairs, care homes) are increasing. I have seen estimates where it says that almost 80 percent of the UK's population suffers from some kind of back issue.

So I say that yoga teachers are the ones who can help in a very positive way. We can't cure conditions but we can ensure that people are aware of ways of minimizing common ailments. There is nothing in the body that cannot repair itself if fed properly, exercised, rested and cared for.

My own story is a case in point. Study the facts, study the logic behind what I had to do to allow the body to heal. The irony is that almost all of the advisors I saw, especially in the medical field, were themselves suffering from some form of back pain. I could not believe that I was seeking help from people who themselves were not well. I seriously wanted to be well, and yes my teacher appeared.

Chapter Two

Six postures to realign, repair and maintain your spine

My intention here is to promote the benefits of yoga through yoga teachers and yoga practioners.

I also intend to introduce a change in the mind of most people in the community who first look at medication as the answer to their conditions. An intentional change and understanding of the use of yoga postures that encourage everyone to consider yoga as a remedial tool.

In the past year or so I have noticed that several of my regular students have been referred to yoga by their doctor or their physio or a chiropractor. This is a good sign and I know that yoga teachers will meet the growing demand.

It is only the yoga teachers and yoga practioners, through their own examples and use of words that people can understand, who can help to increase the number of people enjoying and benefitting from practice of yoga.

You are already a very good example, having picked up this book, of what a body (and mind) can achieve through regular yoga practice. Yoga teachers know that their students also want the same and teachers will always remind them WHY they do yoga.

Whichever way yoga teachers articulate their comments and

instructions, they are giving everyone an opportunity to gain the same benefits that they get out their own practice.

A very small percentage of any given population in the western world do or practise yoga. That means a vast majority of the population is not getting any specific benefits of yoga.

What is the reason for such a small percentage of people in the community doing yoga? Apart from the myths surrounding yoga, there is a lot of misunderstanding of what yoga is about. Yoga teachers will need to work for many more years to dispel the myths.

Practise of yoga brings energy in to the body. This is best understood and observed when a typical yoga session is followed by some pranayama (breathing) and then a few minutes of relaxation.

You will find that the whole class is not only quiet but several of the students may even fall asleep. This is a response from the body due to absence of stress, plenty of warmth and energy in the body, and because there has been a focus on postures and breathing, the mind also becomes quiet, (mindfulness).

So compare yoga with energy coming in to the body, to gym exercises as energy going out of the body.

I am only talking of Hatha yoga as I know it. My style of yoga is driven by precision, holding of postures for a few breaths and to work the body, It has no comparison to fast-moving yoga.

I have no opinion on any of the other styles of yoga, except to say that I personally do not go for the more vagarious yoga simply because I do not see the benefits, and personally did not experience any benefits.

I do not consider a "high" after a yoga session as a good result. The high is due to a whole range of hormones and enzymes circulating in the body. Yes, cortisols and endorphins are body's natural production, but adrenaline is not conducive to good health and a quiet mind.

The aim of a yoga practice is to allow the body to relax and mind to become quieter.

Remember, we are aiming for a stress-free body. Less stress means less chances of any unwanted conditions developing in the body.

The following pages gives the reader a six-posture yoga practice. The postures are specifically selected and modified to strengthen the muscles around the whole of the spine. The postures also build strength in muscles that support the whole body.

I am always very happy to help with explanations and more text, should you wish for further information, simply email me: sam@ samraoyoga.com

Cervical Spine, Thoracic Spine and Lumbar Spine

Cervical spine. The neck spine is made up of 7 vertebrae with the skull balanced and supported by a strong ligament called the nucal ligament. The cervical spine is surrounded by muscles, tendons and ligaments. There is also a large measure of fascia and all the arteries, veins, capillaries, lymphatic system nodules and a whole range of nerves radiating out towards the shoulders and to the arms.

Thoracic spine. Made up of 12 vertebrae and providing support to ribs at the back. Again, large measure of muscles that allow the spine to move in various directions including rotation. Arteries, veins and capillaries provide the means to maintain good health, strength and flexibility.

Lumber spine. Consists of 5 large vertebrae and often referred to as L1 to L5. Majority of problems with lower back reside within these 5 vertebrae. Each one is capable of moving in every direction and also has a wide range of rotation movement. There are lots of muscles supporting this area and when these muscles are not used properly there is almost always pain!

Posterior and Anterior Chain of Muscles

The back of the body, posterior, is an integrated series of muscles, ligaments and tendons. Once you get to know and become aware of the range of muscles and the work they do, you can begin to introduce postures that enable stretching, flexing and real supportive strength building of these muscles.

Posterior chain

The chain starts at the back of the heel; that is where the soleius muscle starts and works its way up to the back of the knee. On top of the soleius is the gastrocnemius which is best described as the calf muscle.

The backs of the thighs are where we have 5 strong muscles generally called the upper hamstrings, then 3 layers of glutes, then the large latissimus dorsi all along the back.

The big back muscle is just under the skin. Then you are between the shoulder blades and to the back of the neck, which is the trapezius muscle.

This is the posterior chain and when worked properly it supports the spine very well.

Anterior chain

This chain starts from the fronts of the feet, up along the front and sides of the shin up to the knees. Then it goes on to the quadriceps (thigh) muscles.

There are 4 strong muscles in the thighs: vestus latralis, rectus femoris, vestus medialis and the sartorius.

Up the front of the hips (hip flexor) along the belly (obliques, transverse abdominis and rectus abdominis), pectoral muscles and all the front of the neck muscles.

Basic starting postures for ALL body types

Posture 1: Virasana (Hero Pose)

Start your practice with this basic posture, sitting on the backs of your heels. A simple posture that allows the fronts of the feet to stretch. Knees are flexed to their maximum. Arches of the feet are stretched. Calf muscles are squeezed and the deep vein and its valves are activated with physical pressure. Hip joints are in a relaxed position. The spine is in its upright position. The head is balanced on top of the spine.

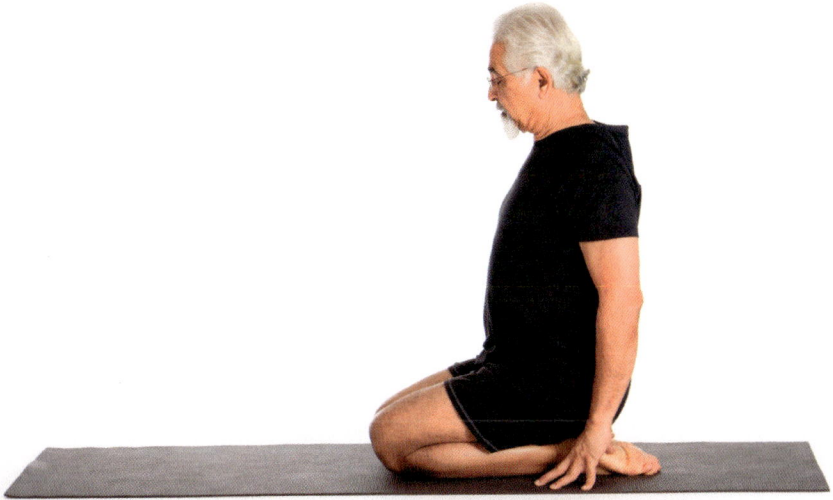

Sitting on the backs of your heels.

There will be many challenges in this starting posture, ranging from simply not being able to sit on the backs of the heels, feeling pain in the knees and perhaps even cramps in the feet. This is not uncommon. Use one or more blocks to sit on. Blocks are placed lengthways between the feet. It may take time for the muscles and tendons to stretch and over time students will find it relatively easy to sit in virasana. Teachers can encourage and sell the benefits. All day the feet and knees get used but very rarely are they allowed to stretch.

For those who find this difficult, despite the supports, give yourself permission to come out and tuck the toes on the mat and then sit back on the heels. Sometimes this is also not so easy. Use 3 to 5 blocks so you get to experience the posture and feel potential, long-term benefits.

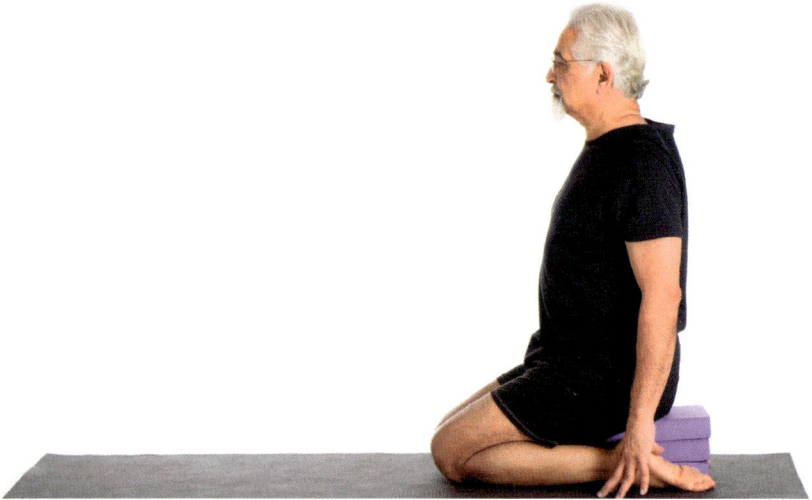

Use blocks between the feet, if fronts of feet are too tight.

For those students who are comfortable to sit on the heels, go a bit further into Balasana (child posture). Hold your feet. Then take a deep breath in and slowly fold forward on an exhalation. Put your forehead on the mat, or close to the mat, and then focus your shallow breathing into the back of the ribcage. Feel the movements of the ribs at the back.

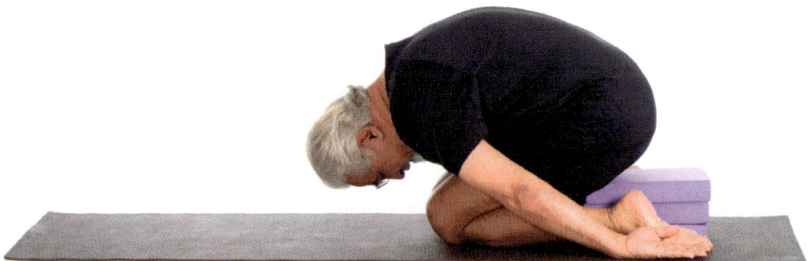

Folding forward to stretch the spine.

Come back up to sitting on blocks, if you are using them, and sit upright and focus on breathing, ribcage opening sideways, towards the elbows.

Posture 2: Virasana (Hero Pose) Variation

Now go into stretching the whole spine. Sitting on the backs of the heels (or on blocks) open the knees wide, hands are on the knees or thighs. Exaggerate the arch in the lower back by using hands on the knees to help and lift the collar bones.

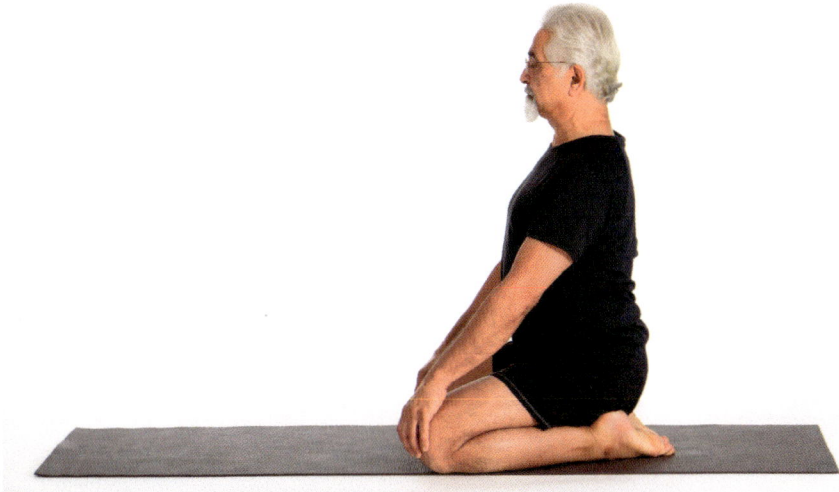

Virasana - preparing to stretch the whole spine.

Then again, on exhalation, fold forward and allow the forehead to rest on the mat. Keep bum on the heels or near the heels. Again, this is not so easy for some. It is ok if the bum lifts away from the heels. Stretch both hands forward to the top of the mat and use the fingers to creep hands forward. The posture now allows the whole of the spine to stretch.

From this starting and warm up postures, you are now ready to go through the four posture sequence for the spine. My suggestion is that you develop your own way, slowly, for the whole session.

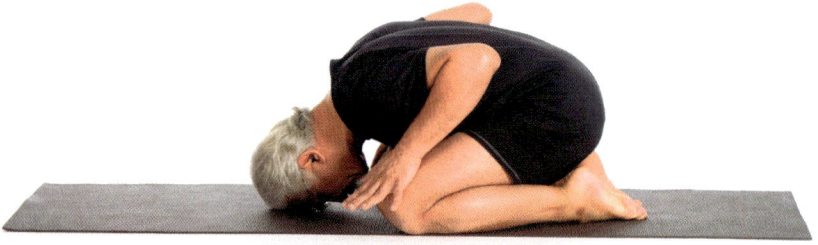

Start slowly. Head may or may not touch the mat.

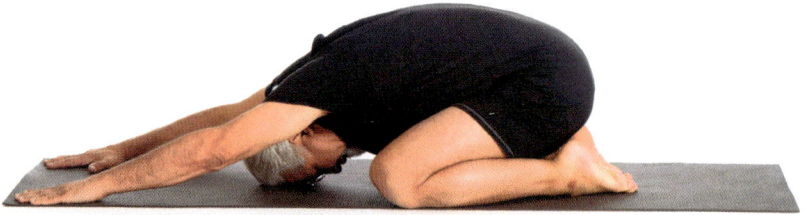

Stretch arms forward and 'pull' head away from hips.

Posture 3: Marjariasana Variation (Thread the Needle)

This posture enables movement of the spine with and against each vertebrae.

Marjariasana Level 1

This level is for everyone. From complete beginners and first time new students and experienced yogis.

From sitting back on the backs of heels, open the knees as wide as the mat. Then lean forward and place the palms on the mat and directly under the shoulders. Focus on a spot between your palms where your right shoulder will drop to the mat.

Now feed (thread) the right hand, behind the left hand, along the mat/floor until the right shoulder and forehead to rest on the mat.

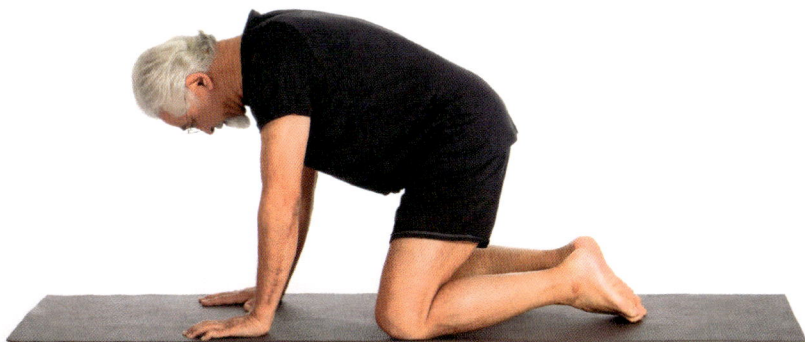

Start in a 'silver back' posture. Knees wide, big toes touching, palms under shoulders.

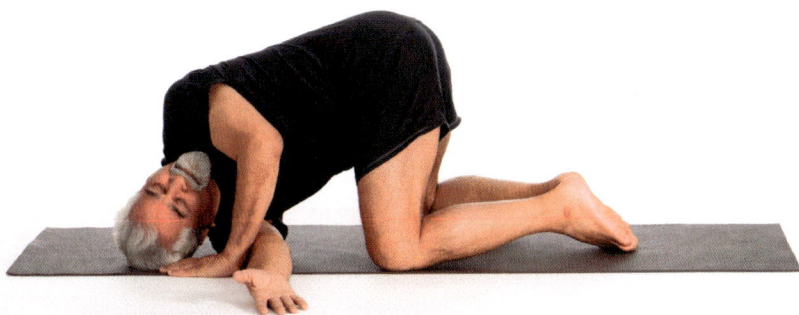

Slowly feeding the arm along the floor to drop the shoulder to the floor.

Only go further if the shoulder is on the mat, if not then hold the posture and come back out to observe and practise until the shoulder is ready to drop to the mat.

Once the shoulder is on the mat, slowly turn your head and bring the chin as close as possible to the left shoulder. The side of the head or even the back of the head will be on the mat. EVERY muscle in the neck is now at work and allowing the cervical spine (neck) to achieve the maximum rotation.

Now lift the left hand towards the ceiling and allow the fingers to slowly disappear beyond the peripheral vision.

This is as far as you want to go for your first few attempts.

Marjariasana Level 2

This enables everyone to start to understand how they are going to build upon their own posture. Remember that we are working on moving the spine in a rotating movement and that is what releases all the physical stress in all the muscles around the spine.

Tuck the left toes on to the mat and slowly straighten out the left leg and keeping the left toes on the mat. (Caution: pay attention to the knee that is now starting to bear the body weight. IF there is any negative feedback in the knee COME OUT of the posture).

Now allow the left hand to go towards the floor behind you and gradually build the range of movement until both the shoulder blades are on the mat and back of left palm is on the floor.

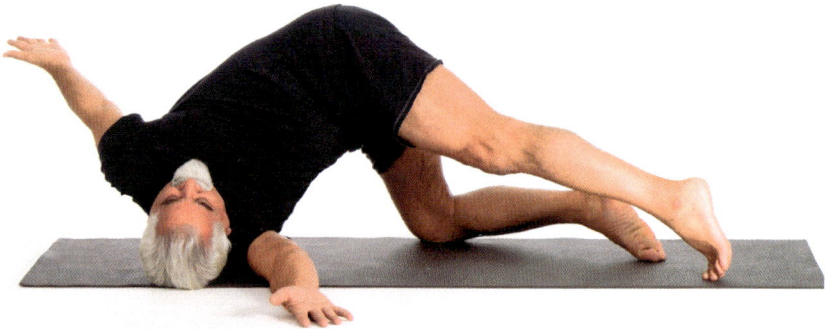

Extending the twist and stretch in this second level.

The entire spine has been twisted along with all the muscles, arteries, veins, capillaries, lymph nodules etc. There is complete range of movement. Level 2 may take several months or years to develop to its full extent.

Come back to sitting on the back of your heels and observe how you feel.

Now repeat the posture on the other side.

Knees as wide as the mat. Lean forward with palms under the shoulders, feed the left hand behind the right until the left shoulder lands on the mat. Turn your head and bring the chin close to the right shoulder, then lift the right hand and allow the fingers to disappear from peripheral vision.

New students come back out, older hands tuck right toes on the mat and straighten right leg and allow the back of the right palm to go towards the floor. Sometimes one side is easier then the other.

Posture 4: Padangusthasana – Supine Variation (Supine Reclined Leg and Lumbar Spinal Twist)

Padangusthasana Level 1

I always encourage use of this posture to all of my students, and especially those with lower back pain and any sciatic nerve related issues.

This posture has proved many times to be very effective for releasing the aches and pains of daily office life. Minor aches and lack of the lower back arch can be corrected over time.

I simply call this posture a variation on Padangusthasana. A supine version. Start with practising level 1.

Lie on your mat, facing the ceiling, spread the arms wide, in line with the shoulders, (you need room on either side of your mat) knees bent with both feet planted on the mat. Feet are hip-width apart. Feel the contact of the shoulder blades with the mat. Try and keep this contact of shoulder blades with the mat, throughout the posture.

Place the right foot on top of the left knee. On an exhalation, twist at the spine and take the right knee towards the left elbow until the right toes are ready to touch the floor.

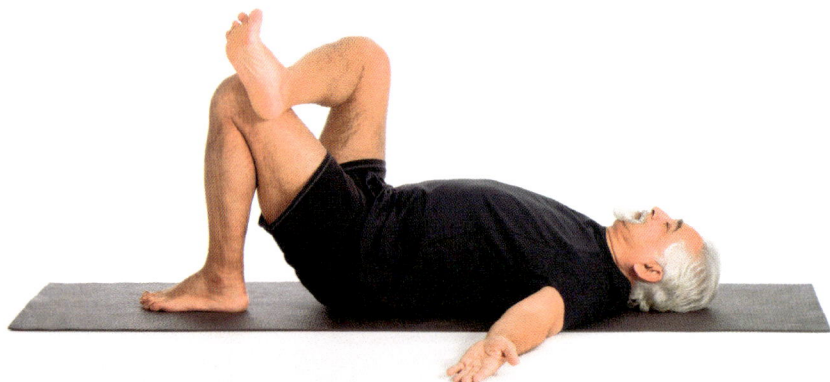

Starting: figure of four with right foot on top of left knee.

(Sometimes if you have a tight midriff or if you are bulky in the core, take heart...I can assure you that it will be a while and after several attempts, that the right toes will touch the floor. It may take many months but it will happen.)

When the toes touch the floor, reach with the left hand and help the right knee to go closer to the floor.

There is already quite a stretch on the right hand side of the hip. The tibial band is being stretched, and the origin of the tibial band is the one that lets you know its being stretched. This posture is very effective at helping ease aches and pains in lumber spine and hips.

The right shoulder blade tends to lift up. Ease up on pushing down the knee and allow the right shoulder blade to go back on the mat.

(Caution: especially if there is anyone who has had breast cancer and has had surgery, they will have tight pectoral muscles that require release over long periods of practice.)

For those who have no challenges in their upper front body they are now feeling the benefits of the stretch of the pectoral muscle. There will be a stretch all along the front of the chest, under the armpits and right to back of the upper arm. Stretch and move the lymphatic system. This is truly the area where "moving water does not decay" comes in at its most beneficial.

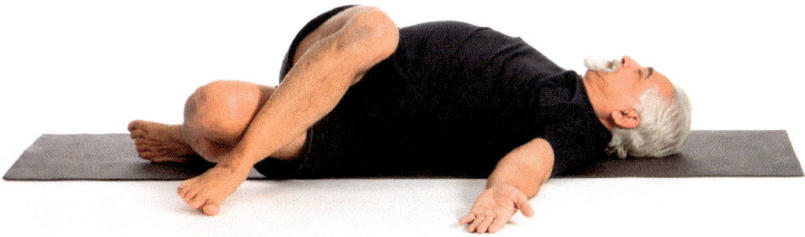

Twisting to the left until foot touches the floor.

The lower back is now in a full twist. The key is to be patient and hold the posture for at least 10 to 15 breaths. This ensures that ALL the muscles around the lumber vertebrae are fully stretched/flexed.

This movement of the lumber vertebrae with and against its neighbour promotes movement of the cartilages between the vertebrae.

The range of movement will be different in every person. It is therefore up to you to guide yourself. Ideally you are building up the range of movement where the right knee is touching the floor, the right shoulder blade is on the mat and back of the right hand is on the floor, in line with the shoulder.

This posture releases all the physical tension/stress that builds up during the day in this area. Depending upon the kind of posture you hold during your working day, the resulting hold of the posture will be different.

A person driving a car all day, a person sitting at a desk most of the day, and young mothers carrying children on their hips, etc. each one will experience different kind of ache in their lower back.

Release the posture, come back to the centre and prepare and do the other side.

Padangusthasana Variation Level 2

Go for level 2 once you are happy with the range of movement in level 1.

With the right knee being pressed towards the floor and the right shoulder blade almost touching the mat, engage your awareness to your right fingers and open the fingers as wide as you can.

This begins to stretch the nerves. The nerves to control the movement of the fingers and the arm originate from the cervical spine, the vishudhi chakra region. The nerves travel along the arms to the fingertips. You will start to feel the stretch of the nerves.

Begin to guide your their right arm along the floor towards 10 o'clock, 11 o'clock and eventually to 12 o'clock position.

As you study and develop this part of the posture and allow yourself to slowly build the range of the arm movement, you will see the benefits.

Stiff shoulders will begin to release. Rotator cuff muscles at the front and back of each shoulder begin to stretch and allow a wider range of movement. The most important benefit is that the lymphatic system in the upper part of the body is allowed to move to its maximum.

Release the posture, come back to the centre and prepare to do the other side, starting with level 1.

Padangusthasana Variation Level 3

Continue to build upon level 2, then take this posture further. Bring the right arm back in line with the right shoulder. Turn your head to face to your left.

Straighten out the right leg and support the right leg from under the right knee, palm supporting the back of the knee, the elbow on the mat/floor supporting the leg.

This is already introducing a stretch in the hamstrings and once the knee is locked in then start to bring the right toes in line of sight.

This is a wonderful stretch for the hamstrings and also an extended movement for the right hip-joint and the muscles close to the lumber spine (longissimus and quadratus lumborum).

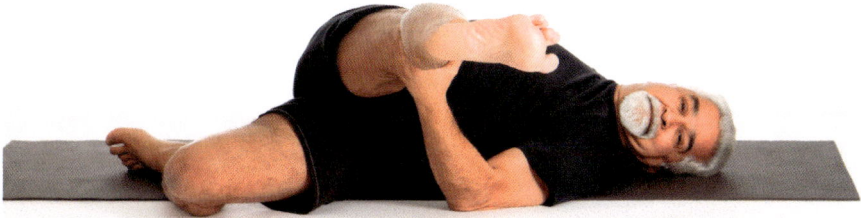

Extending the stretch along the right leg and along the hip and spine.

Release the posture, come back to the centre and prepare to do the other side.

Start with level 1 on this side, going into level 2 and then to level 3 and build upon the posture by holding for increasing number of breaths.

Posture 5: Utkatasana (Sitting on an Imaginary Chair)

This is a strong standing posture and it will activate and work the whole posterior chain of muscles. Work this posture with your awareness. Tendons and muscles from the heels to the back of the head will work in concert.

Stand at the centre of your mat. Feet are hip-width apart. Raise your hands above your head, palms facing in.

Slowly push your bum back, tuck your chin in and look at your toes.

Begin to bend at your knees a little and go as if you are preparing to sit on an imaginary chair behind you. You will see your knees starting to come towards the toes.

PUSH the knees back over the heels and keep pushing the bum back and down. You will start to feel the glutes engage and work. The backs of the legs will be working.

Push the bum back, keep bending the knees but keeping the knees over the heels and raise your hands up towards the ceiling. Look straight ahead and hold for 5 to 10 breaths.

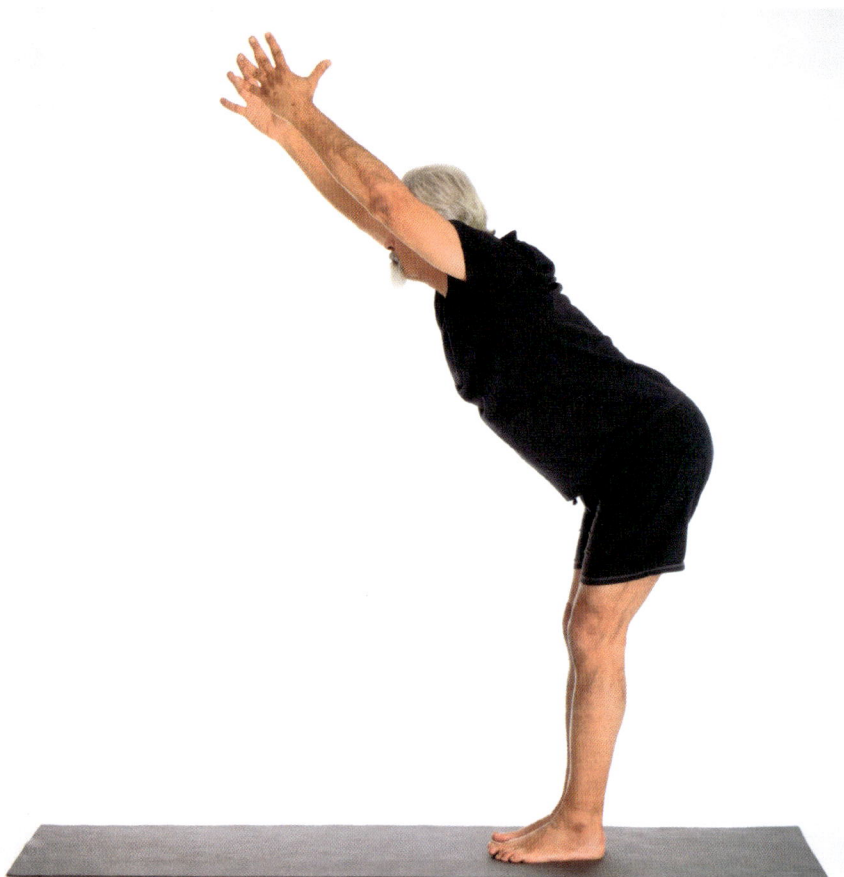

Keep knees over the heels – *activate posterior chain of muscles.*

Build the posture slowly. FEEL the glutes tightening, feel the whole posterior chain muscles working.

Posture 6: Virabhadrasana (Warrior One)

This is another strong standing posture and the one that really builds the strength around the spine.

Stand towards the very back of your mat with the length of your mat in front of you.

Put your hands on your hips. Come up on the ball of the right foot. Step forward with the left leg, go at least a leg length forward. Place both hands on the left knee.

Check that the left knee is over the left heel. Move or creep the left foot forward to make sure of this alignment.

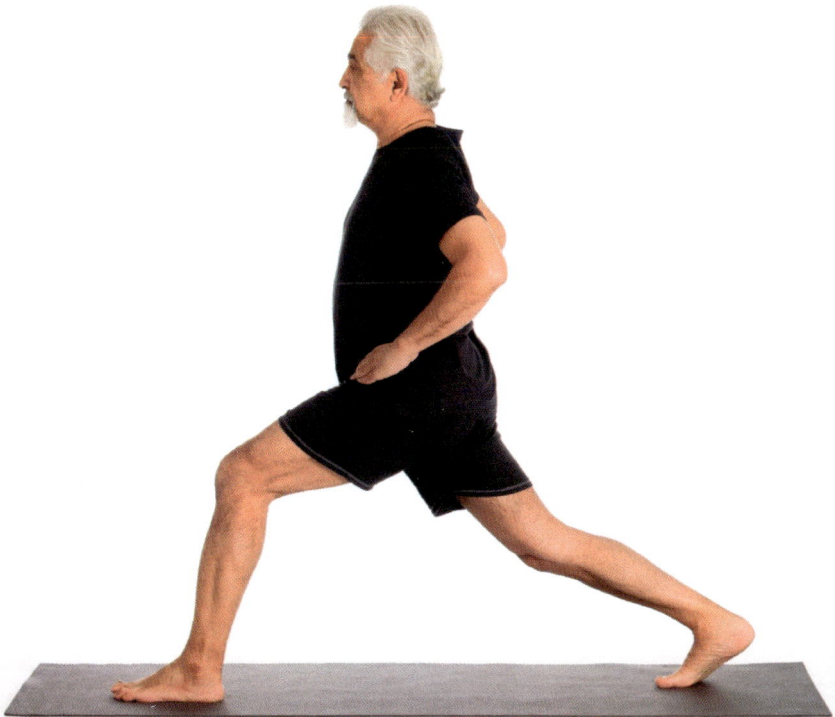

Start with this posture; balance and ensure front knee is over the heel.

Push the torso upright and then lift both the arms up to the ceiling. Both sets of toes are pointing forward. The heel at the back is off the mat. Lean back to also activate the obliques and the core muscles. Hold for 5 breaths.

Slowly fold forward, fingers in pyramids, place the fingers either side of the left foot and slowly straighten out the left leg and allow your forehead to go towards the left knee. Hold for 5.

Look at the floor, bend the left knee and then step the right leg forward and come up. Tip-toe back towards the back of the mat and repeat the posture on the other side.

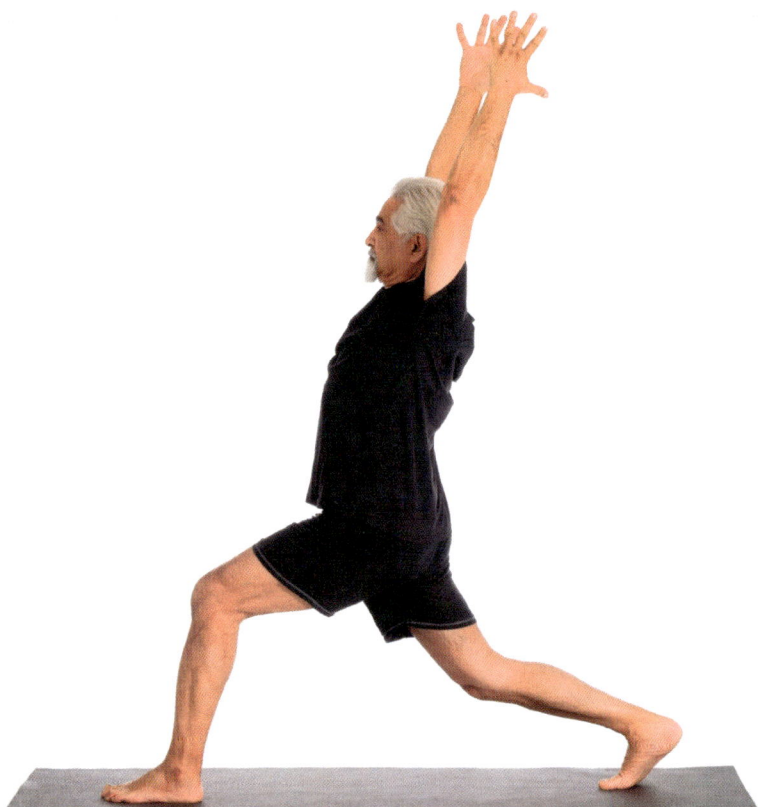

Raising the arms up and arching the back to work both posterior and anterior chains of muscles.

Chapter Three

Nutrition

The second part of the rehabilitation programme called for continuation of supporting the body with a full spectrum of vitamins and minerals. I would strongly recommend this to anyone who wants good support for the body at cellular level.

Daily Nutritional Intake

Intake of very high quality supplements ensures that each and every cell in the body is being fed properly, every cell is supported with what it needs to ensure its health.

Table 1 outlines various supplements containing vitamins (shown in Table 2) and minerals (shown in Table 3). These supplements are developed with specific ailments in mind.

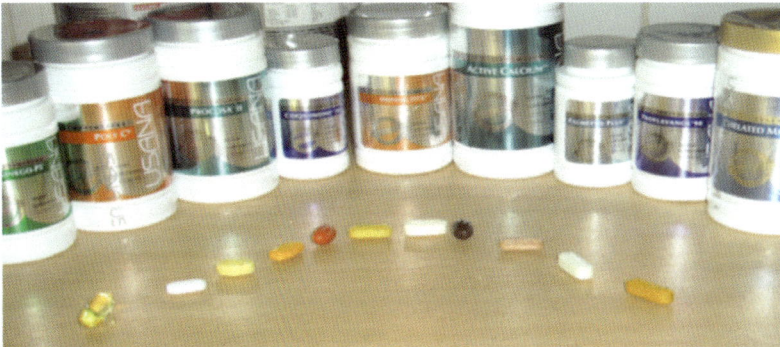

These are high quality supplements and my daily dose.

Table 1 - Supplements

Item	Type	What for
1	Antioxidants	Vitamins
2	Minerals	Chelated minerals that are bio-available
3	Active calcium	Calcium that the body recognizes as food
4	Palmetto plus	Specifically for prostate gland – Lycopyn (men only)
5	Coq10 (30)	Cardiac muscles and nerves
6	Ginko	Brain tissue function
7	Proflavinol 90	Anti-inflammatory
8	Hepesil dtx	Liver detox
9	Poly c	Organic vitamin C
10	Biomega 3	Omega 3, 6 & 9 oils
11	Procosa II	Glucosomine for joints

Table 2 - Vitamins

Item	Quantity	What for
Vitamin A	15000 iu	Healthy skin, protect from infections, immune system booster, against cancer, night vision.
Vitamin C	1800mg	Immune system, bones, skin, strong joints, anti-oxidant, anti-stress, hormones, detoxify pollutants.
Vitamin D	450 iu	Makes strong bones by retaining calcium.
Vitamin K	60µgm	Controls blood clotting.
Vitamin E	450 iu	Antioxidant, helps use oxygen, prevents clots, thromboses, athrosclarosis, skin.
Vitamin B6	27mg	Protein digestion, hormone production, anti-depressant, controls allergies.
Vitamin B12	60µgm	Essential for homosystene balance.
Calcium	1300mg	Healthy heart, nerves, controls muscles, maintains acid-alkaline balance.

Item	Quantity	What for
Magnesium	1000mg	Strong bones and teeth, muscle relaxant, heart muscles, cofactor in many enzymes, nerves.
Rutin	14mg	Anti-cancer, anti-thrombotic, cyto protective, strengthens capillaries.
Quercetin	6mg	Anti-inflammatory, anti-tumor properties, helps prostate function.
Boron	1.32mg	For prostate. Micro-nutrient, cell-wall builder.
Silicon	9mg	Necessary for enzymes and hormones to function.
Lycopene	8mg	Most potent carotenoid antioxidant, comes from tomatoes, high concentration in prostate gland.
Soy Isoflavins	25mg	Isolflavins are polyphenolic compounds that are capable of exerting oestrogen-like effects.
Iodine	225µgm	Iodine deficiency causes goiter.
Zinc	40mg	Component of over 200 enzymes, healing, controls testis, ovaries, stress buster, helps nervous system, brain. Constant energy.
Selenium	400µgm	Antioxidant, reduces inflammation, stimulates immune system, healthy heart, male reproductive organs.
Copper	6mg	Electrolyte and catalyst for a large number of hormones to function.
Manganese	7.5mg	Healthy bones, cartilage, nerves, active in over 20 enzymes, stabilizes blood sugar, insulin production, brain function.
Chromium	300µgm	GTF Glucose tolerance factor, bloodsugar balance, protects DNA, RNA, essential for heart function.

Item	Quantity	What for
Molybdenum	50μgm	Helps rid of uric acid, helps teeth, detoxify blood from petrochemicals, sulphites.
Vanadium	30μgm	Electrolyte and catalyst for a large number of hormones to function.
Thiamin B1	27mg	Energy production, brain function, helps to use proteins.
Riboflavin B2	27mg	Repair and maintain skin, sugar & fats to energy, regulate body acidity, hair, nails, eyes.
Folate	1000μgm	Red blood cells formation, essential for brain function.
Niacin B3	40mg	Energy production, balance blood sugars, lowers cholesterol, brain function, skin.
Biotin	300μgm	Helps use of essential fats, healthy skin, hair, nerves.
Glucosomin	1000mg	Joint lubrication
Turmeric	250mg	Powerful antioxidant.
Phosphorus	800mg	Bones, teeth, builds muscles, DNA, RNA, maintains Ph, metabolism, energy.
Potassium	2000mg	Byproducts in and out of cells, fluid balance, relaxes muscles, insulin, heart function.

Conclusion

The results, after over 3 years since my first MRI and X-rays I have no more pain.

I do my daily personal yoga practice and teach yoga. I feel and I know I am fully fit.

My spine was examined again by Dr Carraway early in 2015 and he declared that the lumber spine vertebrae were all back to their normal position. The vertebrae have all almost aligned back.

The stenosis is still there and occasionally I feel the sciatic nerve along my left leg and down to my left foot.

It does not stop me doing what I like.

Chapter Four

What I did
to change my
condition

My programme of rehabilitation concentrated in two specific areas: yoga postures and nutrition. I was to continue to use vitamins and minerals to support my body.

My journey to enable my spine to return to where it was, so that I can continue to do most of the sports I enjoyed and to continue to build upon my yoga seems a long one, but very worth while.

I take great pleasure from my activities:
- Walking for miles.
- Cycling even more.
- Teach between 6 to 10 yoga classes per week, including 1-2-1 sessions
- Organizing and running 3 (1 week long) yoga retreats per year,
- Doing at least 3 CPDs (to help yoga teachers and students to keep on developing their yoga) per year.
- Running my Yoga Teacher Training school where I have an average of 10 trainee teachers every year.
- Do 3 to 4 workshops and 1 exhibition per year.
- Visiting yoga teacher at several gatherings in London.
- And I am always looking to go to more gatherings and be a student or a teacher.

The following are some of the 24 different yoga postures that I practised for my spine and I also teach to my clients who have and are suffering from a bad back.

These postures enabled me to build the muscle structure around the spine area that was damaged, and I only teach what I do myself.

Halasana (Plough Posture)

This is a strong posture that stretches the entire posterior chain

DO NOT do these postures without having guidance from an experienced yoga teacher.

DO the postures suggested in Chapter Two and then you find a yoga teacher who is ready to support and guide you through some or all of the postures in this chapter.

of muscles from back of the head right through to the back of the heels. It also opens the lumber vertebrae at the back and closes them at the front. I needed to do this posture to maintain muscle integrity, once the muscles were strong.

Marjariasana (Thread the Needle)

There are 5 levels to this posture and the objective is to enable

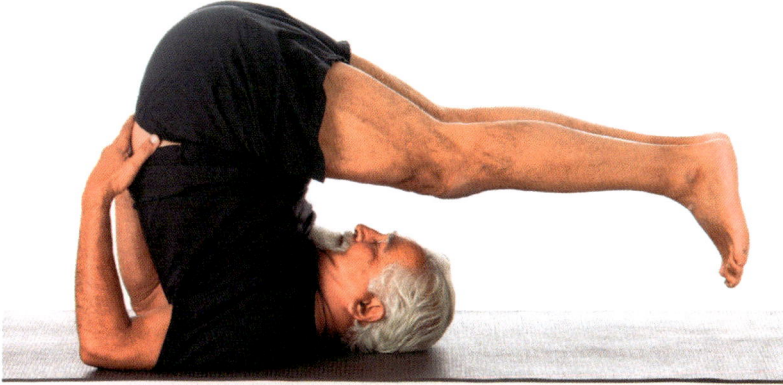

rotation of each vertebrae with and against its neighbour, thus stretching and building more strength in all the muscles around the spine.

Padangusthasana – Supine Variation (Legs and Lumber Spine Twist)

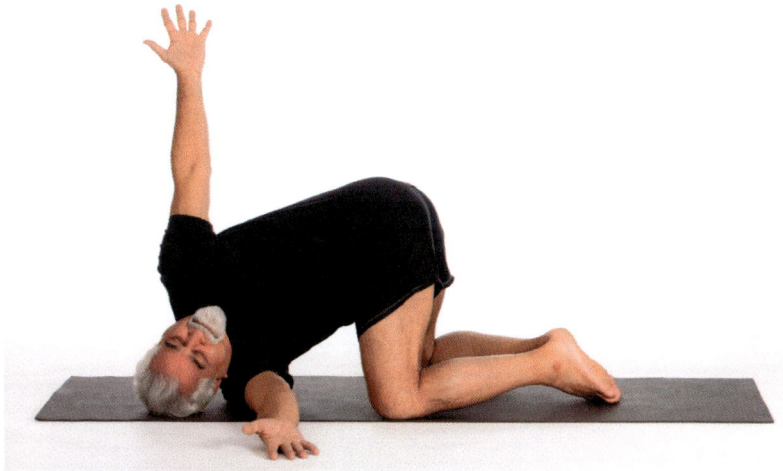

There are 3 levels to this posture and the objective is to rotate all the lumber vertebrae and also include all the supporting muscles that include the glutes, upper hamstrings, lower hamstrings. The best benefit of this posture is that it helps to release the sciatic nerve.

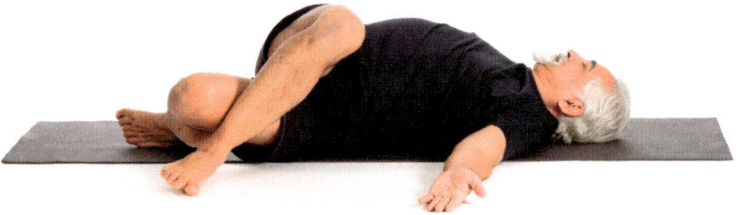

Utkatasana (Sitting on an Imaginary Chair)

This is level 1 of the posture that helps to build the strength in the entire posterior chain. There are several levels to this posture and eventually this posture helped the most to work on bracing the lumber spine. A strong series of postures with excellent results.

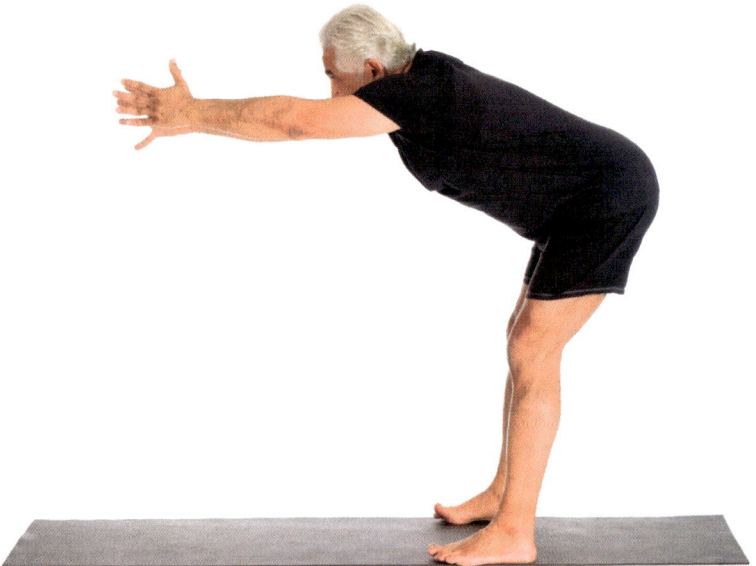

Virabhadrasana 1 Variation (Warrior 1)

Warrior postures are real strength builders and this is a variation that is again the one that has delivered strong muscles of the back and the front. The entire spine in this posture is worked, both in movement and in also strengthening the muscles around the spine.

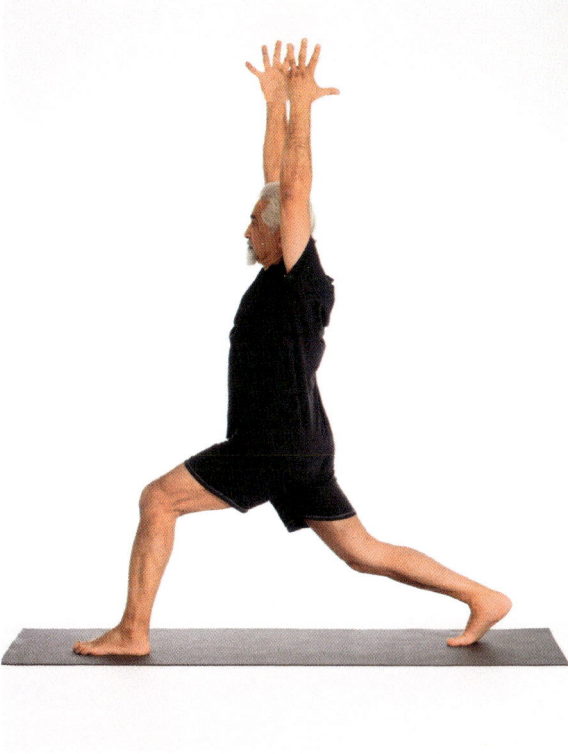

Ardha Adho Mukha Vrksasana (Half-Handstand)

Half-handstand in a way is an easier version that everyone can do safely. The result will be the same but may take longer.

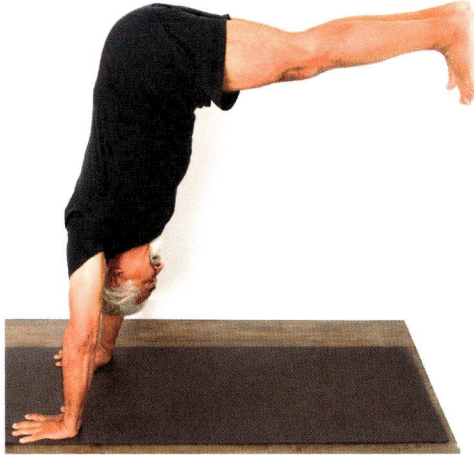

Adho Mukha Vrksasana (Handstand)

Handstands have long been recognized to help build the strength in both the posterior and anterior muscle chains. The arch in the lower back is stretched to its maximum and helps to release a lot of the physical tension in the area.

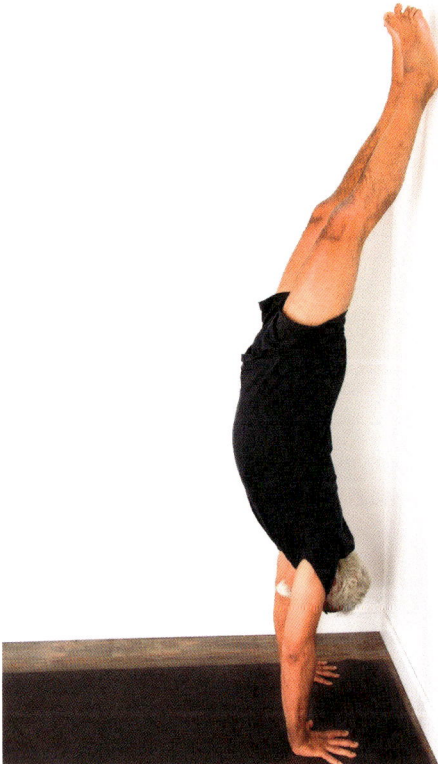

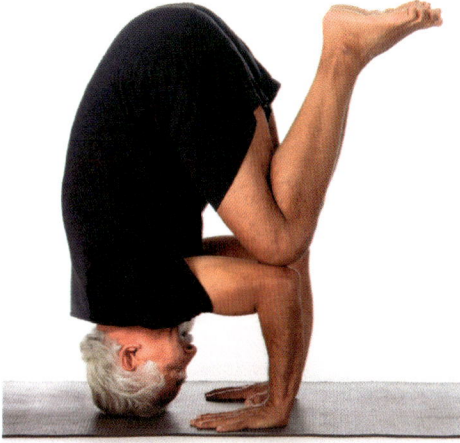

Bakasana Variation (Crane or 3-Pointed Headstand)

Builds strength in all the layers of muscles along the spine.

Develops control over psoas and illiacus muscles as the legs are raised into this 3-pointed headstand.

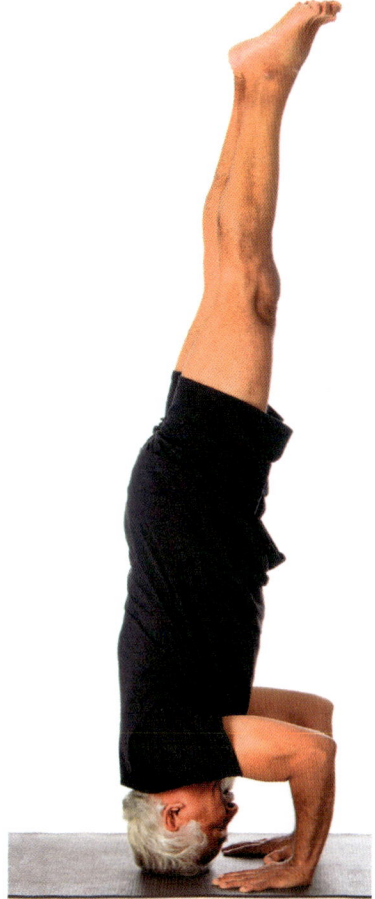

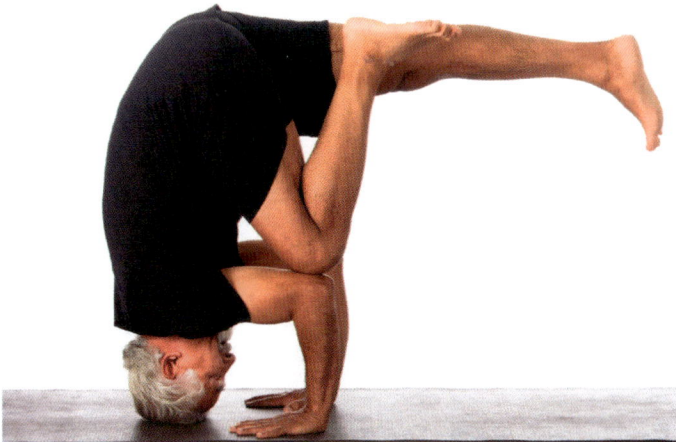

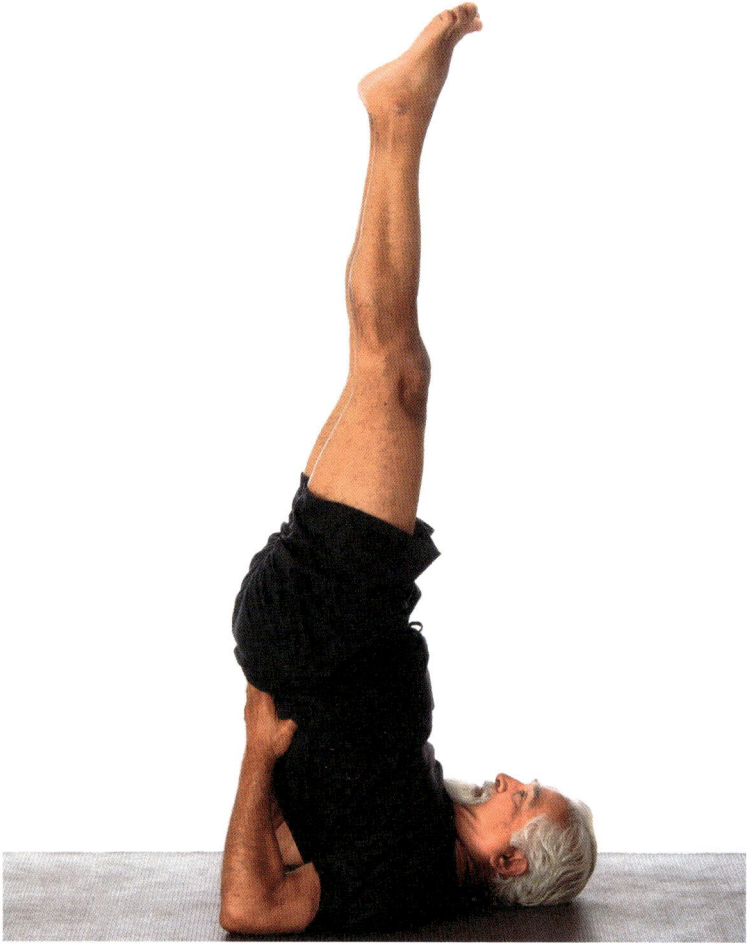

Salamba Sarvanghasana (Supported Shoulder Stand)

With the spine supported well the core body muscles of the anterior chain gain strength and flexibility, leading to supporting the lumber spine.

Variation on the 3-pointed headstand. Spine is straight and all the front and back muscles are being strengthened.

This posture must not be done if there are issues in the wrists or neck.

Usine Bali Yoga Sling for inversions
(not recommended without supervision)

Bali yoga sling is a support that enables the whole body to be used while safely supported. The purpose for me was to use the upper body weight to stretch the spine.

Inversions are always energising and I have found the sling to be a very valuable addition to my yoga postures for maintaining my spine.

It supports the hip and allows the spine to stretch, using upper body weight.

This is one of the best ways I know of continuing to build core strength, stretching the spine and allowing the body to heal itself.

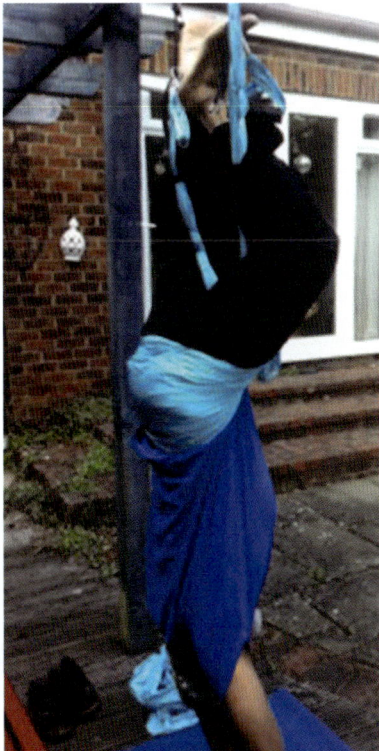

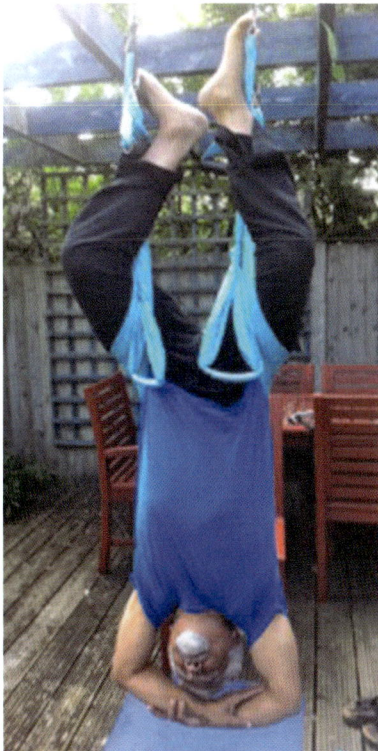

Conclusion

This is the story of Sam Rao.

An old squash-playing days injury eventually manifested into serious lumbar spine issues.

Sam came across his teacher, Dr Carraway, when he needed help to sort out his back problem. Sam is against any medical interventions in back ache or back pain issues.

Chapter Two explains what Sam did to realign and repair his spine, and continues to maintain the health of his spine through continued daily yoga practice.

Sam recommends that everyone could do the postures shown to ensure that the strength and flexibility of the whole spine is maintained throughout life.

Index

Printed in Great Britain
by Amazon